AROMATHERAPY

A guide for home use

by Christine Westwood

Published by Amberwood Publishing Ltd
Guildford, England.

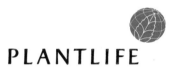

PLANTLIFE

The Natural History Museum, Cromwell Road, London SW7 5BD

Registered Charity No. 328576

Amberwood Publishing supports the Plantlife Charity,
Britain's only charity exclusively dedicated to saving wild plants.

ISBN 0 9517723 0 9

Cover design by Howland Northover

Printed in Great Britain

CONTENTS

Christine Westwood

Christine Westwood has her own Aromatherapy practice in London. She trained with Robert Tisserand in 1982, and was a founder Director of The Tisserand Aromatherapy Institute.

At the Findhorn Foundation in Scotland, she worked in an herbal apothecary, where her attention was drawn to the healing power of plants.

She also trained in Art Therapy, Counselling, Nutrition, Reiki and Hypnotherapy which she combines in her natural healing practice.

During her work as a qualified accountant she became interested in researching and developing strategies for coping with stress. As a stress management consultant she has helped individuals from many organisations achieve their maximum potential.

She is a frequent contributor to the media, and her work has been included in several books and publications on Aromatherapy. She holds regular workshops on Aromatherapy and other natural healing techniques.

Christine would like to thank her friends, family and colleagues who encouraged her to produce this book, in particular Michael Mauger who helped with the important task of editing the book.

Introduction to the Guide

'Aromatherapy – A Guide for Home Use' is an Introductory guide to Aromatherapy for the general public. It provides an easy-to-use reference section of essential oils and their applications, for conditions commonly encountered.

The book is not intended as a substitute for consultations with a qualified Aromatherapist. Additionally, where symptoms persist beyond a reasonable period always consult a doctor, or your Professional Aromatherapist who can liaise with the medical profession.

Interest in Aromatherapy has grown substantially in the last few years. It is hoped that the reader by becoming aware of the conditions that may be helped by the essential oils, will wish to regard the oils as a common addition to the family first aid kit. Hopefully once curiosity has been aroused, there will be a wish to pursue the ensuing interest.

Note to Reader

1 | What is Aromatherapy?

i) Aromatherapy oils, and how they are used

Aromatherapy is the use of organic essences of aromatic plants for healing and the maintenance of vitality.

The essences, or 'essential oils' as they are commonly known, are extracted from a wide variety of plants, and are very concentrated. For example it takes the petals from about 30 specially cultivated roses to produce one drop of Rose essential oil and several kilos of lavender to produce a small bottle of essential oil.

Each oil has its own unique healing properties and fragrance. One essential oil may contain over one hundred different chemical constituents. These oils in their natural state have been found to possess a powerful 'synergy' i.e. the therapeutic quality of the unadulterated natural oil is more effective than a synthetic, partially reconstituted equivalent.

The essences are volatile and will evaporate without trace if left open to the air. They do not dissolve in water.

Several oils are often used in combination to promote healing on different levels – physical, mental and emotional.

There are several ways of using the oils, all of them very pleasant: massage, bathing, compress, inhalation (never use them orally).

They work by the absorption of minute quantities of the oil through the skin, and also through inhalation of the aroma.

ii) History and development of Aromatherapy

Smell has always been one of the most powerful and perhaps one of the most instinctual of all our senses. It must have guided our earliest ancestors in their choice of foods and medicinal herbs. Burning different woods on their fires they could have experienced the stimulating effect of Rosemary, and the restoring effect of Sage.

Knowledge of how to make use of the beneficial effects of aromatic plants developed gradually. By 3500BC, the priestesses of the Egyptian temples were burning gums and resins, such as Frankincense, to clear the mind. The Romans used essential oils for massage, and aromatic herbs within the home.

In 17th century England, pomanders made of Oranges and Cloves were used to ward off the Black Death. Great herbalists such as Culpepper used essential oils such as Peppermint and Rosemary as an integral part of their medicine.

The 19th and 20th centuries saw the development of chemistry and the creation of synthetic drugs. Their widespread use overshadowed the use of more traditional remedies.

Interestingly it was a chemist, the Frenchman Rene Gatefosse, who in 1937 coined the word 'Aromatherapy'. He was working in the laboratory of a perfumery when he badly burnt his hand. He plunged it into the nearest bowl of liquid. It happened to be essential oil of Lavender. The hand healed with exceptional speed and virtually no scarring. As a chemist, Gatefosse realised that the healing and antiseptic qualities of this pure essential oil of Lavender were manifestly much greater than any of the synthetic equivalents available to him. He subsequently researched into the healing properties of other essential oils. Another Frenchman, Dr Valnet, added to this research whilst working as a medical surgeon in the Second World War. Medical supplies were short, and the essential oils proved to be a very effective alternative in many cases. The work of Rene Gatefosse, Dr Valnet and several other eminent researchers helped in the scientific validation of Aromatherapy.

Since the war Aromatherapy has continued to develop in different ways in different countries. In France there are over 1500 medical doctors who have trained in Aromatherapy. In the UK its growth has been part of the 'complementary medicine' movement. Today it is used by thousands of people from all walks of life, including Royalty.

iii) Aromatherapy in the UK

Aromatherapy as it has developed in the UK, is based on an holistic approach, which seeks to encourage health on all levels.

For example if a woman has arthritis, Rosemary, Juniper or Chamomile might be considered to help the physical aspects of the condition. Her feelings would also be taken into account. Is she suffering from resentment, or anger about her condition? If this was the case, different oils would be chosen to help with these psychological aspects of her state of health. The chosen oils would act as a catalyst to promote healing on all levels.

Another important part of the holistic approach is the encouragement it gives for people to help themselves and take responsibility for creating their own health. Home use of Aromatherapy is a very practical way of doing this.

iv) Aromatherapy – an aid to stress management and vitality

Proper use of the oils helps promote a more balanced lifestyle. There is less likelihood of succumbing to everyday illness and the effects of stress.

A balanced state of mind promotes vitality and better ability to cope with potentially difficult events, such as a boardroom meeting or a visit to the dentist.

Use of Aromatherapy can also stimulate the immune system, avoiding the 'run-down' feeling that can often lead to colds or flu.

2 | How essential oils are obtained

i) Sources of essential oils

Essential oils are obtained mainly by distillation, and a few by solvent extraction. Other methods such as expression have been used, but are generally too labour intensive to be cost effective. The essential oils are obtained from different parts of the aromatic plant: –

Essential Oil	Source of the Essential Oil
Fennel	Seeds
Jasmine	Flowers
Orange	Fruit (Peel)
Lemongrass	Grass
Geranium	Leaf
Ginger	Root Tuber
Sandalwood	Wood

ii) Distillation

Large vats are filled with the selected part of the plant which is processed by steam distillation. The essential oil is separated from the cooled condensed water producing, for example, Lavender essential oil and Lavender water.

Some plants may produce several oils as different sections of the plant are processed, e.g. the Orange tree gives: –

Essential Oil	Source of the Essential Oil
Orange	Peel
Pettigrain	Leaves
Neroli (Orange Blossom)	Flowers

iii) Solvent extraction

Solvent extraction is used for fragile flowers such as Jasmine, where the heat and pressure used in distillation would destroy the essential oil. The flowers are placed in layers of wax and solvent to macerate and are renewed daily. Subsequently, they are put through a centrifuge and distilled at very low temperatures.

This process can take up to 20 days to complete, and oils obtained in this manner are understandably expensive.

The result of this process is called an absolute. Essential oil of Rose is also produced by this process as well as by distillation.

3 | Purchase and storage of essential oils and base oils

i) Purchase of essential oils

In order to benefit from the healing properties of the oils, it is vital to purchase them from a reputable supplier who takes care to ensure high standards. Before accepting a batch, a sample will have been tested, using gas chromatography, to see whether the characteristic 'signature' of the pure essential oil is evident. The word 'natural' on a bottle's label does not always guarantee purity. It is sensible to check that the description states 'pure essential oil'.

Buy the oils in small quantities as you need them, replacing them as required.

ii) Storage – how to care for the essential oils

Keep the essential oils in dark glass bottles in which they are supplied. Blends may be kept in similar bottles, (12-20mls is a good size). These may be obtained from a chemist for a reasonable cost. Plastic containers are not suitable for storage. The oils are very powerful and will damage them.

Make sure the top of the bottle is always securely shut, as the essential oils are very volatile.

Store them in a cool environment away from direct light.

Always ensure that they are out of reach of inquisitive children.

iii) Storage – how long will they last?

Most essential oils will keep for up to two years.

In particular Citrus oils such as Orange and Grapefruit may only be effectively used for up to six months. Then they will go cloudy through oxidation.

On the other hand there are a few essential oils which improve with age, rather like some good wines. These are often the oils which originate from plants which have taken a long time to mature, e.g. Sandalwood and Frankincense. There is even a market for vintage Frankincense!

Blended oils remain effective for up to three months if stored in a cool place such as a refrigerator.

iv) Purchase of base oils

It is important that high quality base oils be chosen with the essential oils.

Extra virgin cold pressed oils should be used. These come from the first pressing. Later extractions use heat or solvent processes which destroy the trace minerals and vitamins found in the oils. Similarly avoid mineral and baby oils.

Sweet almond is a popular and excellent choice for a base oil.

Almond oil diluted with 10% of Avocado or Wheatgerm (unless the user is allergic to wheat) is good for people with particularly dry skin. Other carrier oils include Grapeseed, Apricot Kernel, Peach Kernel, Olive, Soya, Sunflower Seed and Sesame Seed. Jojoba, which is a wax, may also be included in a blend.

4 | General cautions, children and special cases

NEVER USE NEAT ESSENTIAL OILS DIRECTLY ON TO THE SKIN. NEVER USE THEM INTERNALLY.

i) Babies, infants and children

Babies and infants should only be treated with the oils recommended in the paragraph immediately below. They, and to a lesser extent children, require much smaller amounts of the oils than adults to obtain effective results. Use these oils as indicated in the reference section.

Babies 0-12 months	One drop of Lavender or Roman Chamomile a) compress b) room fragrancer c) dilute one drop in 15ml of Sweet Almond oil for i) massage ii) bathing
Infants 1-6 years	One – three drops of Tea Tree, Lavender or Roman Chamomile used as above.
Children 7-12 years	Use as for adults but half the number of drops of essential oils.
Children 12+ years	Use as directed for adults.

ii) Pregnancy

USE THE ESSENTIAL OILS IN HALF THE STATED AMOUNT AT THIS SPECIAL TIME.

Stimulating essential oils and those which have an emmenagogic effect, i.e. help bring on periods, should not be used during pregnancy.

Basil, Clove, Cinnamon, Hyssop, Juniper, Marjoram, Myrrh, Sage and Thyme, should not be used during the nine months of pregnancy.

Fennel, Peppermint, and Rosemary should be avoided during the first 4 months of pregnancy, because of their stimulating effect, but are acceptable after this period.

iii) Eyes

Keep essential oils away from the eyes. Should an accident occur, wash the eyes with plenty of water and seek medical advice.

iv) Homoeopathic treatment

If receiving Homoeopathic treatment, consult your homoeopath, and avoid the following essential oils: Black Pepper, Camphor, Eucalyptus and Peppermint. They may nullify the Homoeopathic preparations.

v) Sensitivity and allergies

a) Allergic reactions
People with allergies, including allergies to perfume, may well be helped by professional Aromatherapy. The aromatherapist will recommend the essential oils for home use.

b) Sensitivity
Occasionally a person's skin may be sensitive to a particular oil (usually the more stimulating ones), causing irritation. It will generally disappear within the hour. Plain Sweet Almond Oil, smoothed on the affected part, will help the irritation to subside.

Sometimes women find skin sensitivity increases just before their period, or at ovulation. This is due to hormonal changes in the body.

If sensitivity occurs, refrain from using the particular oil for 10 days. Then, if you wish to use it again, dilute to one quarter of the original amount, and test on a small area of the skin. If no reaction occurs, you can continue to use the oil in the diluted amount.

Certain oils are best administered by a qualified Aromatherapist: Cinnamon, Clove, Hyssop and Sage.

5 | Methods of using the essential oils

i) Massage

Massage has been found to be the most effective way of using the essential oils.

For the purposes of massage, the oils are blended in a base oil (see instructions on blending).

Massage of the hands and feet is an excellent way to keep in good health. All the reflex or zone points for the body are stimulated by this method. This helps balance the body's energy flow.

Before considering home massage, it is recommended that you take a basic course. There are many good introductory massage courses available. Find a course with a qualified teacher who is also an experienced practitioner.

ii) Bathing

Bathing is the next most effective way of using the oils. There are two alternative ways of proceeding:

diffusing up to 5 drops of essential oils
OR
diffusing up to 5ml of a blend.

This method is good if you have sensitive or dry skin, or wish to preserve a suntan.

PROCEDURE

a) Run a bath of warm water (not hot or the oils will evaporate too quickly).
b) Add up to 5 drops of either essential oil or 5ml of the blend.
c) Agitate the water.
d) Relax for 10-15 minutes minimum.
e) Avoid splashing in the eyes.

It is safe to use the bathing method everyday. The warm water assists the absorption of the oils. You may not be aware of the effects immediately, perhaps not until the next morning after the sound sleep which such baths often promote.

As you notice changes in your condition, you may wish to vary the oils according to the new indications. The body will benefit from the different properties of the essential oils.

If your condition doesn't begin to change after a reasonable amount of time, it is wise to consult a qualified Aromatherapist in conjunction with medical attention if necessary.

iii) Inhalation

Inhalation is very useful for relieving congestion, easing catarrh and soothing the respiratory tract. The age old method of covering the head with a towel and inhaling the vapour from Eucalyptus and Camphor still holds good today.

PROCEDURE

a) Boil 2 pints of water and pour into a bowl.
b) Add 10 drops of an essential oil or a combination of essential oils.
c) Agitate the water.
d) Put a towel over the head. Close the eyes and inhale the vapours for a few minutes at a time, for up to 10 minutes or as long as is comfortable.
Repeat several times a day if required.
   A facial steamer may be used instead of a bowl with 3-5 drops of essential oils.

iv) Compresses

Follow first aid instructions for the use of compresses and disperse 1-2 drops of essential oil into the water. The material should be gently laid on the surface of the water to attract the film of essential oil. The compress can then be placed on the affected area in the normal way.

v) Scalp treatments

A range of scalp conditions, including dandruff, respond well to the use of an essential oil blend.
   This method can also be used to assist in clearing lice from the scalp and has the advantage of being pleasant to use.

PROCEDURE

a) Ensure that the eyes are well protected.
b) Prepare the chosen blend (proportionally less for children) and massage into the scalp.
c) Leave the mixture on the head for half an hour to two hours.
A plastic cap will help absorption. Always supervise children as they may pull a loose fitting cap down over their face. Bathtime is a good time for a scalp treatment as heat aids absorption.
d) To remove the blend: massage in neat shampoo initially, then add water and shampoo in the normal way.

vi) Room fragrancers

There are several ways of using essential oils to produce a wonderful fragrant atmosphere in a room.

a) Essential oil burners

Essential oil burners are obtainable in many health food shops and from some suppliers of the oils.
   A small reservoir at the top of the burner is filled with water. This is heated by the flame from a nightlight placed inside the burner. Up to 5 drops of neat essential oil may be sprinkled on the water. This gradually evaporates, filling the room with the aroma. For example Lavender produces a relaxing atmosphere which can help with insomnia. Rosewood is soothing for tired, grumpy children who don't want to go to bed.
   During illness, the use of a room fragrancer can help to protect the health of the rest of the family. The 'aroma' inhibits infection by airborne bacteria such as cold and flu viruses. This has been put to good test in several hospitals and clinics. This method can also ease breathing in many chest conditions and may help asthmatics reduce their need for inhalants.

b) Light fittings

Put a few drops of neat essential oil on a cold light bulb or use a special attachment for the bulb. The fragrance will gradually permeate the room as the warmth of the bulb vaporises the essential oil.

c) Humidifiers

A saucer of water with a few drops of neat essential oil placed on top of a radiator will act as a vaporiser and humidifier at the same time.

vii) Handkerchief or tissue

Put one or two drops of neat oil onto a handkerchief or tissue and inhale when required. This method is useful for travelling and when other methods are not convenient.

viii) Perfumes

Make up a blend as directed and use as you would a perfume. Frankincense and/or Sandalwood make excellent fixatives for your blend.

6 | How to use the reference guide with examples

Choosing the right essential oils from the physical index is quite straightforward.

Choosing from the psychological index is more of an adventure. When exploring the new 'territory' of physical and psychological balance it helps to have the open-mindedness of 'Alice in Wonderland'. The journey can be very exciting.

i) Guidelines

1. Using the Physical Reference Index is a good way to become familiar with the use of essential oils. This index can be used on its own, see Example I, or in conjunction with the Psychological Reference Index, see Example II.
2. Each person's condition is unique. He/she needs to find out which oils and blends work best for them.
3. The oils are powerful catalysts. Respect the indicated maximum amounts.
4. You may wish to use less than the indicated amounts. A more dilute blend can sometimes be just as effective.
5. Use the oils to gently stimulate the body's natural healing ability.
6. The oils may sometimes work a little slower than conventional remedies. It takes several hours for them to be absorbed into the body's system.
7. Use the Essential Oils Guide frequently to become familiar with the unique properties of each oil.
8. The oils are non-addictive and non-toxic.
9. If conditions persist beyond a reasonable time, it is wise to visit a qualified Aromatherapist. A well trained Aromatherapist can liaise with the medical profession if necessary.

ii) Guide to the Reference Section

The reference index is divided into three sections:

a) guide to the essential oils.

It gives a brief introduction to the properties of each oil, and a 'keyword' which describes its overall character. The physical and psychological conditions for each oil are listed under each oil and cross-referenced with the other two indexes. At the bottom of each individual oil's section are symbols describing the cautions for its use.

b) index of the physical conditions, the indicated oils, and symbols for suggested methods of use.

c) psychological conditions, the indicated oils, and symbols for suggested methods of use.

The reference guide also contains examples: –
Example I   – Using the Physical Reference Index
Example II   – Using both the Physical and Psychological Reference Indexes

Example III — Making up a blend
Example IV — Achieving a balanced blend
Immediately preceding the reference sections is a key to the symbols used in them.

iii) Example I: Using the Physical Reference Index
A woman has bad circulation.

PROCEDURE
1. Check the cautions section.
2. Refer to the Physical Reference Index for 'bad circulation'. Rosemary — BM is given.
3. Consult the symbols key to find B = bathing and M = massage.
4. Choose the method of using the oils. Bathing with diffused oils might be the choice in this case.
5. Follow the procedure for bathing using up to 5 drops of diffused essential oil.

iv) Example II: Using both the Physical and Psychological Reference Indexes
A man has sprained his ankle playing his favourite sport.

PROCEDURE
1. Follow normal first aid procedures. Assess the seriousness of the injury. If necessary go to the doctor or the casualty department of the hospital. If home first aid is applicable: —
2. Check the general cautions section. If no cautions apply: —
3. Look in the Physical Reference Index — Lavender and Chamomile oils are indicated. C for compress is indicated as the advised method of use.
4. Later in the day the man may wish to have a bath with a combination of Chamomile and Lavender. See bathing instructions in the methods section.
5. Consider the psychological factors. Talking with a friend or partner can help highlight the reasons for the injury and any possible psychological factors such as:
Was he feeling impatient?
Did he forget to warm up? Is this a bad habit?
6. Looking in the Psychological Index he will find that for 'Impatience' Lavender is indicated (in this case it is recommended for both physical and psychological aspects of the condition). For the release of old habit patterns Rose is indicated. BMR are given as possible methods of use. He chooses B for bathing.

v) Making up a blend
To make up a blend use up to 4 different oils in the base oil of your choice.

PROCEDURE
a) Dilution
1. Ascertain the volume of the bottle in millilitres. Often it is written on the bottle.
2. Divide the number of millilitres by two. The answer gives the number of drops of essential oil you need to add to the base oil. This achieves the recommended ratio of 2.5% essential oil to 97.5% base oil.
If you want to make up a 12ml bottle of the blend you will therefore need to add up to 6 drops of essential oil to the base.

If you want to make up a 20ml bottle of blend you will need to add up to 10 drops of essential oil to the base.

b) Achieving a balanced blend

Fragrance is a subjective experience. It's important for the person who is using the blend to find the aroma balance that instinctively seems right for him or her.

The fragrance of certain oils is particularly strong. These oils need to be used in smaller amounts so that they do not dominate the blend.

Examples are Camphor, Eucalyptus, Peppermint and Tea Tree. The fragrance of other oils such as Jasmine, Rose and Neroli, though not so obviously strong, are very pervasive and could also dominate a blend.

One drop of the above oils is all that is usually needed in a blend.

vi) Example III – Making up a blend

A woman has a tension headache. She is anxious and worrying about the future because her husband is likely to be made redundant.

PROCEDURE for choice of oils

1. Check the caution section.
2. Look in the Physical Reference Index: Lavender is indicated for the headache (tension).
3. Look in the Psychological Reference Index: Bergamot is indicated for anxiety. Sandalwood is indicated for worry about the future.

Because her skin is dry she has chosen the method of using a blend in the bath, with Sweet Almond oil as the base.

PROCEDURE for blending

a) Fill a clean 12ml bottle with Almond oil.
b) Calculate the maximum amount of essential oils to be added, i.e. 12ml divided by 2 = 6 drops of essential oil.
c) Check the intensity of each oil's aroma by smelling it. In this case they are of similar intensity so add 2 drops of each to the base oil.
d) Replace the top and gently shake the bottle to mix the blend.
e) Follow instructions on bathing using a blend.
f) Store the rest of the blend in a cool place or the fridge (but not the freezer!) for future use. The blend may be kept for up to three months.

vii) Example IV – Achieving a balanced blend

A recently bereaved woman with arthritis wishes to massage her hands.

PROCEDURE

1. Follow steps one to three above.
In the Physical Reference Index: Juniper is indicated (for swelling), Lavender is indicated (for pain).
In the Psychological Index: Rose is indicated (for grief).
2. She wants to make up a 20ml blend. Twenty millilitres divided by two = 10 drops of essential oil – the maximum number of drops to be added to the blend.
3. She adds one drop of Rose (one of the heady oils).
4. She adds three drops of Juniper (it smells stronger to her than Lavender).

5. She adds four drops of Lavender. These 8 drops may be sufficient to produce the pleasing aroma of a balanced blend.

6. She may however, add further drops of either Rose, Juniper or Lavender, up to the maximum of 10 drops total, if this would make the blend more agreeable.

Keeping a notebook of the blends you make and the results they give will help you to build on your growing experience.

7 | Symbols Key

B   BATHING
C   COMPRESSES
H   NOT SUITABLE IF RECEIVING HOMOEOPATHIC TREATMENT
I   INHALATION
M   MASSAGE
N   MAY BE USED NEAT WHERE INDICATED IN EMERGENCIES
    (Lavender and Tea Tree only)
P   NOT SUITABLE/RESTRICTED USE DURING PREGNANCY
R   ROOM FRAGRANCE BURNER
S   SENSITIVE SKIN
U   DAB WITH A COTTON BUD
★   A COUPLE OF DROPS ON A PILLOW AT NIGHT
○   USE A COUPLE OF DROPS ON A HANDKERCHIEF
□   SCALP TREATMENT

✕   NOT TO BE USED FOR:
    b – babies   0-12 months
    i – infants   1-5 years
    c – children 6-12 years
    Over 12 as adults

CAUTIONS – SEE GENERAL CAUTIONS SECTION AND THE ESSENTIAL
OIL GUIDE FOR SPECIFIC GUIDANCE FOR CAUTIONS AS APPLICABLE
TO EACH OIL.

Keywords give an indication of a primary quality and the 'character' of the essential oil described. They act as a useful guide when making a selection.

8 | Guide to the essential oils

BASIL ~
Key word: *Clearing*

Ocimum basilicum

Distilled from the well known culinary herb, oil of basil is an excellent aromatic nerve tonic. It clears the head and gives the mind strength and clarity. It is an effective aid for exam nerves.

Use in small amounts. It mixes well with Geranium, Bergamot and the Citrus oils.

Physical conditions
Headache with congestion
Sinus congestion
Fainting

Psychological conditions
Lack of concentration
Mind tired/exhausted, short attention span
Memory poor
Listless
Mental stimulation
Lack of discipline

Cautions: ✗ b i c P S

This essential oil is best administered by a qualified Aromatherapist.

BERGAMOT ~
Keyword: *Uplifting*

Citrus bergamia

Obtained from the rind of a small orange-like fruit native to Italy, it is valuable for depression, anxiety and skin care. Its light, uplifting fragrance blends well with other essential oils.

Physical conditions
Boils
Depression – PMT
Herpes
Psoriasis
Travel sickness – fear

Psychological conditions
Anxiety
Depression
Despondency
Negative thoughts
Monday morning feeling
Obsession
Regret
Confidence, lack of
Shyness
Stress

Cautions: ✗ b c i: Do not use within 3 hours of going out in the sun or using a sunbed, as pigmentation of the skin may be affected.

BENZOIN ~
Keyword: *Soothing*

Styrax benzoin

Benzoin is a resin and is one of the ingredients of 'Friars Balsam'. Its warming, soothing and penetrating qualities are useful for conditions which are slow to heal.

Physical conditions
Blisters
Chapped and cracked dry skin

Psychological conditions
Loneliness
Sadness

Cautions: ✗ b i

BLACK PEPPER ~
Keyword: *Penetrating*

Piper nigrum

From Malaysia. It is one of the oldest known spices, being used in India over 4,000 years ago. The oil has a hot stimulating effect. It dilates local blood vessels making it very useful for aches and pains and as an aid for digestion.

Physical conditions
Constipation
Flu
Muscle aches
Fever
Sickness, stomach pains

Cautions: ✗ b i c H

CAJUPUT ~
Keyword: *Focusing*

Melaleuca leucadendron

Useful for respiratory conditions, it will also relieve a fever. Its penetrating aroma is useful for breaking through old habits and focusing in the present.

Psychological conditions
Compulsiveness/obsessions/habits
Cynicism
Disorientation
Clarity
Memory
Procrastination

Cautions: ✗ b i c

CAMPHOR ~
Keyword: *Piercing*

Cinnamomum camphora

A powerful oil. Useful for conditions where the person is cold. Capable of piercing through the thoughts of a wandering or worried mind.

Psychological conditions
Daydreaming
Nerves: worry about the future

Cautions: ✗ b i c P H and Epileptics

CARDAMON ~
Keyword: *Expansion*

Elettaria cardamomum

A spicy warming essential oil. A good remedy for digestive problems. Where there is a focus on internal problems, it expands the person's awareness, the warmth bringing more openness.

Physical conditions
Colic
Indigestion

Psychological conditions
Confusion
Selfishness

Cautions: ✗ b i c

CEDARWOOD ~
Keyword: *Composing*

Juniperus virginiana

Cedarwood has a pleasant, smokey odour. It has a long history of use by the Egyptians. When inhaled it has a composing effect. It is useful for catarrh and for an oily skin.

Physical conditions
Asthma
Bronchitis
Dandruff
Oily skin

Psychological conditions
Stress
Scattered thoughts

Cautions: ✗ b i c P

CHAMOMILE MOROCCAN ~

Ormenis multicaulis

It is often confused with Chamomile Roman. It is not a substitute, as it belongs to a different plant family. References in this guide refer to Chamomile Roman.

Cautions: ✗ b i c

CHAMOMILE ROMAN ~
Keyword: *Soothing*

Anthemis noblis

Roman chamomile is one of the most useful essential oils. It is anti-inflammatory and thus soothing in its action. This essential oil may be safely used with children in the stated dilutions.

Physical conditions
Bedwetting
Boils
Chilblains – itchy and burning
Colic
Dermatitis
Eczema
Hot flushes
Nettle rash
Rheumatoid arthritis
Sensitive and inflamed skin
Sprains, joints and tendons
Swollen joints

Psychological conditions
Impulsive
Overactive mind
Restless mind
Tantrums
Worry

Cautions: None

CINNAMON BARK ~

Keyword: *Fevers*

Cinnamomum zeylanicum

Traditionally used as a remedy for many digestive problems, it is a powerful skin irritant and should be used with care. As a room fragrancer it blends well with Orange and Clove oil.

Physical conditions
Shivering cold
Flu-like symptoms
Cautions: ✗ b i c P S
This essential oil is best administered by a qualified Aromatherapist.

CLARY SAGE ~

Keyword: *Euphoric*

Salvia sclarea

Distilled from the whole plant, it has a warm, nutty scent. A very good muscle relaxant and a key essential oil for PMT.

Physical conditions
Addiction
Exhaustion
Insomnia – physically overtired from
overwork
PMT

Psychological conditions
Claustrophobia
Compulsiveness
Depression
Dreams – recurrent
Hostility
Hyperactivity
Insomnia
Listlessness
Negative thoughts
Obsession
Over-analytical
Overwork – mental strain
– nervous exhaustion
Relaxation
Restless with exhaustion
Stress
Sulking

Cautions: ✗ b i P

CLOVE ~

Keyword: *Pain reliever*

Eugenia caryophyllata

Obtained from the flowerbuds of a small evergreen tree from Madagascar. Traditionally associated with the relief of toothache and a powerful antiseptic.

Physical condition
Toothache
Cautions: ✗ b i c P S
This essential oil is best administered by a qualified Aromatherapist.

CORIANDER ~
Coriandrum sativum

Keyword: *Appetite stimulant*

A sweet smelling spicy essence, stimulating and refreshing in the bath.

Physical conditions
Lack of appetite
Cautions: ✗ b i

CYPRESS ~
Cupressus sempervirens

Keyword: *Astringent*

This oil is obtained by distillation of the leaves and cones of the tree, which grows in the Mediterranean region. The astringent properties of this essential oil make it very effective in a foot bath.

Physical conditions
Asthma
Bedwetting
Bronchitis cough
Cellulitis
Chestiness
Dry cough
Dandruff with an oily scalp
Haemorrhoids
Muscles: aid to convalescing
Heavy periods
Nosebleeds
Urination – frequent
Cautions: ✗ b i

Psychological conditions
Jealousy
Sluggishness
Too talkative

EUCALYPTUS ~
Eucalyptus globulus

Keyword: *Respiratory system*

One of the tallest trees in the world, the whole tree exudes an aromatic odour, imparting a healthy atmosphere to the regions where it is grown. Widely used as an inhalant and chest rub, it contains powerful antiseptic properties.

Physical conditions
Asthma
Bronchitis
Catarrh
Colds – flu-like symptoms
Colds – runny nose
Colds – headaches
Congestion – catarrh
Cystitis – temperature with respiratory [1]
tract
Sinusitis – headaches and relief of
sinusitis
Cautions: ✗ b H

FENNEL ~

Keyword: *Normalising*

Foeniculum vulgare

Cultivated by the Romans, the herb is traditionally used in cooking to combat obesity. It was said to convey strength, courage and longevity.

Physical conditions
Abdomen bloated
Wind
Appetite excessive
Cellulitis
Colic
Flatulence
Indigestion
Nausea from overeating
Overweight

Cautions: ✗ b i P

FRANKINCENSE ~

Keyword: *Rejuvenating*

Boswellia thurifera

Also called Olibanum, it is extracted from the gum of a small North African tree. It has a warm, spicy scent. It has been prized for centuries, and it is a helpful aid to meditation.

Physical conditions	**Psychological conditions**
Abscess weeping	Apprehension
Acne scarring	Bereavement − prolonged grief
Cold − likes hugging fires for comfort	Claustrophobia
Cracked and weeping skin	Courage
Haemorrhoids	Fear
Nosebleeds	Insecurity
	Irritability following a fright
	Nerves − worry about the past
	Nightmares
	Panic attacks
	Paranoia
	Perseverance in difficult circumstances
	Security
	Self criticism
	Stability
	Supportive
	Undisciplined

Cautions: ✗ b i

GERANIUM ~

Keyword: *Balancing*

Pelargonium odorantissium

Also known as Rose Geranium the oil is pale green in colour and comes from Madagascar. The scent is fresh, floral and sweet. It is useful for most skin conditions and has a stimulating effect on the lymphatic system. It blends well with most other essential oils. It tends to balance extremes whether on the physical or emotional level.

GERANIUM ~ *continued*

Physical conditions
Change of life
Dermatitis
Eczema – skin sensitive to touch
Hormone balancing
Lice
Periods irregular
PMT
Pregnancy
Skin blotches/dry/normal
Cautions: ✗ b

Psychological conditions
Attachment
Mood swings
Rigidity
Too extrovert/introvert

GINGER ~
Keyword: *Digestion*

Zingiber officinale

Produced from the root by steam distillation. It should be used in small amounts at all times.

Physical conditions
Arthritis
Bilious attack
Cold symptoms
Flu – early stages
Intense cold
Cautions: ✗ b i c S

Psychological conditions
Self-acceptance
Self-awareness

GRAPEFRUIT ~
Keyword: *Releasing*

Citrus paradisi

Grapefruit has a lovely tangy, uplifting aroma. Helpful for ditherers and those who find it easier to stay with the old, rather than decide to follow the new.

Psychological conditions
Bitterness
Clarity
Confusion
Despondency
Envy
Frustration
Indecisiveness
Jealousy
Procrastination
Worry about the past

Cautions: ✗ b i

HYSSOP ~
Keyword: *Stability*

Hyssopus officinalis

Hyssop has the ability to stabilise a condition when used in small amounts.

Physical conditions
Hypertension
Hypotension

Psychological conditions
Grief

Cautions: ✗ b i c P and Epilepsy

This essential oil is best administered by a qualified Aromatherapist.

JASMINE ~
Keyword: *Aphrodisiac*

Jasminum officinale

One of the most expensive essences, often referred to as the King of the flower oils. Jasmine has a wonderful exotic fragrance and makes a luxurious and enjoyable massage oil.

Physical conditions
Childbirth
Flu – early stages

Psychological conditions
Apathy
Aphrodisiac
Detachment
Emotional expression
Fear of coming events
Frigidity
Jealousy
Over-analytical
Rigidity
Sadness
Secretive
Shyness
Stress
Too extrovert/introvert

Cautions: ✗ b i c

JUNIPER ~
Keyword: *Toxin elimination*

Juniperus communis

Juniper oil is distilled from the berries and has many uses. Its main qualities are its blood purifying and cleansing properties.

Physical conditions
Arthritis swelling
Cramps
Cystitis
Hangover
Hayfever
Periods – scanty
Rheumatism
Urination – burning and painful
Water retention

Psychological conditions:
Lethargy
Protection

Cautions: ✗ b c P

29

LAVENDER ~
Lavandula officinalis

Keyword: *Immune system*

Probably the best known of the essential oils. It is a number one choice for the first aid kit at home.

Physical conditions
Abscess
Acne
Antibiotics
Arthritis – pain
Baldness
Bed wetting
Bites
Blisters
Bruises
Burns
Chestiness – dry cough
Chilblains – swollen
Cuts
Cystitis – pain on passing water
Dermatitis
Earache
Eczema
    – Skin cracked and weeping
    – Sensitive to touch
    – Burning and hot
Exhaustion
Headache tension or migraine
Hot flushes
Immune system stimulant
Insect bites
Insomnia
Joints – swollen and painful
Migraine
Nausea
Neck – stiff
Nosebleed
Overwork
PMT
Pregnancy
Skin burns
    – Dry
    – Itchy
    – Weeping eczema
Sprains
Stings
Sunburn

Psychological conditions
Fear
    – following a fright
    – of failure
    – of people
    – stagefright
Hysteria
Hyperactivity
Impatience
Insomnia
Insecurity
Irrationality
Irritability
Mood swings
Negative thoughts
Nerves – worry about the future
Overwork
Paranoia
Relaxation
Restlessness
    – active mind
    – apprehension
Panic attacks
Stage fright
Too extrovert/introvert
Worry

LAVENDER ~ *continued*
Physical conditions *continued*
Tendons – painful
Throat – sore/dry/burning
Tinnitus – sensitive to noise
Travel sickness – restlessness
Cautions: None

LEMON ~   Keyword: *Refreshing*
Citrus limonum
This oil comes from Sicily and is produced from the rind of the fruit. About 3,000
lemons are required to produce a kilo of the essence. It is helpful for banishing warts,
corns and verrucae.

Physical conditions   **Psychological conditions**
Cellulitis   Selfish
Verrucas   Sluggish
Warts
Cautions: ✗ b i

LEMONGRASS ~   Keyword: *Strengthening*
Cymbopogon citratus
The oil has a powerful lemony smell. Often described as resembling lemon sherbert. It
is obtained from a wild grass and is cultivated mainly for the perfume industry.

Physical conditions   **Psychological conditions**
Insect repellent   Boredom
Muscle aches and pains   Lack of interest
                                  Overwork – nervous exhaustion
                                  Sulkiness

Cautions: ✗ b i c

MARJORAM ~   Keyword: *Muscle relaxant*
Origanum marjorana
Best known for its warming qualities. It is good for muscle spasm, aches and strains.

Physical conditions   **Psychological conditions**
Coldness   Hostility
Muscle relaxant   Hyperactivity
                                  Irrational thoughts
                                  Overwork
                                  Mental strain
                                  Muscle tension/relaxer

Cautions: ✗ b i c P

MELISSA ~
Keyword: *Female aspects*

Melissa officinalis

The name means bee in Greek and the smell does attract these insects. Melissa has a beautifully fragrant, lemony, scent; hence its other name of Lemon Balm. It is helpful for allergies and is a gentle tonic. Paracelsus called it the elixir of life.

Physical conditions
Periods – heavy

Psychological conditions
Humility
Nurturing the 'female aspect'
Shock
Worry about the future

Cautions: ✗ b i

MYRRH ~
Keyword: *Resinous*

Commiphora myrrha

Like Frankincense, it is one of the oldest essential oils and has religious significance. Greek soldiers always carried myrrh with them into battles to treat their wounds. It is good for mouth and throat infections.

Physical conditions
Dry cough
Cautions: ✗ b i c P

NEROLI ~
Keyword: *Stress reliever*

Citrus bigaradia

The number one oil for stress and shock, Neroli or Orange Blossom has a truly fragrant aroma.

Physical conditions
Skin – broken veins

Psychological conditions
Bereavement
Disorientation
Fright
Hysteria
Mental strain
Overwork
Restlessness with exhaustion
Shock
Stress

Cautions: ✗ b

ORANGE ~
Keyword: *Radiance*

Citrus aurantium

A warm, cheering oil. Good for those suffering from lack of energy and depression.

Physical conditions
Lack of energy

Psychological conditions
Selfishness
Stubbornness

Cautions: ✗ b

PATCHOULI ~

Keyword: *Pervasive*

Pogostemon patchouli

Widely used in Indian traditional medicine, patchouli has a musky, sweet fragrance which is very persistent. Because of this it is often used as a base for perfumes. It is useful for healing cracked skin and weeping sores.

Physical conditions
Cracked skin
Sores
Overweight

Cautions: ✗ b i

Psychological conditions
Apprehension
Clarity

PEPPERMINT ~

Keyword: *Cooling*

Mentha piperita

Peppermint is used widely in confectionery and medicines. Best known as a remedy for digestive upsets. It makes a good substitute for aspirin. It is also effective against ringworm and scabies. Excellent too for tired feet.

Physical conditions
Aches and pains
Bilious attack
Headache – travel sickness
Itchy skin (one drop only in bath, more may have the opposite effect)
Migraine
Nausea
Neuralgia
Tinnitus nausea
Travel sickness – sensitivity to movement

Cautions: ✗ b i

Psychological conditions
Mental stimulant
Studying

PINE (SCOTS) ~

Keyword: *Invigorating*

Pinus sylvestris

This is obtained from the pine needles. A good inhalant and invigorating in the bath.

Physical conditions
Bronchitis
Respiratory

Cautions: ✗ b i c

ROSE OTTO ~
Keyword: *Cleansing*

Rose centifolia/Rosa damascena

Considered to be the Queen of the flowers. It is an excellent oil for purification on both physical and emotional levels.

Physical conditions
Addiction
Allergies
Hangover
Hayfever
Headache – allergy
Migraine – allergy
PMT – weepy
Skin – mature

Psychological conditions
Attachment
Bereavement – lost in the past
Fear
Grief
Nerves – worry about the past
Regret
Sadness
Self-centredness
Terror

Cautions: ✗ b i

ROSEMARY ~
Keyword: *Stimulant*

Rosemarinus officinalis

A penetrating and stimulating oil with many uses. A good oil for its stimulating effect on both mental and physical levels.

Physical conditions
Baldness
Chilblains
Chilliness
Circulation
Colds – frequent sneezing
Constipation
Dandruff with a dry scalp
Exercise
Hangover
Ligaments painful from overexertion
Migraine
Muscle ache
Shivering from cold
Tendons overexertion
Tiredness

Psychological conditions
Clarity
Disorientation
Indecisiveness
Lethargy
Memory
 – dull
 – bad memory
Mental
 – stimulation
 – calmness
Monday morning feeling
Protection
Sluggishness

Cautions: ✗ b i P ★

ROSEWOOD ~
Keyword: *Freshening*

Aniba roseaodora

Psychological conditions
Apprehension
Daydreaming – excessive
Grumpiness
Stability

Cautions: ✗ b i

SAGE ~
Keyword: *Tonic*

Salvia officinalis

The Latin name for Sage comes from the word Salvation. It was considered instrumental in prevention of illness. Use in small quantities.

Physical conditions
Metabolism stimulant

Cautions: ✗ b i c P S

This essential oil is best administered by a qualified Aromatherapist.

SANDALWOOD ~
Keyword: *Expression*

Santalum album

From Mysore in India, the fragrance is woody and sweet. It is useful for the skin and especially the throat area – traditionally associated with self-expression.

Physical conditions	**Psychological conditions**
Bronchitis	Cynicism
Catarrh	Dread of effort
Carbuncles	Dreams recurrent
Cough – dry	Fear of coming events
Loss of voice	Failure
Cystitis	Humility
Dry eczema	Insecurity
Hoarseness	Intuition
Sore throat	Irritability
Sinusitis	Listlessness
Tinnitus	Nerves, worry about the future
	Perseverance in difficult circumstances
	Security
	Self-centredness
	Sensitivity

Cautions: ✗ b i c

TEA TREE ~
Keyword: *Antiseptic*

Melaleuca alternifolia

The essential oil has a strong medicinal smell. It has many qualities, being anti-bacterial, anti-fungal and a powerful immune system stimulant.

Physical conditions
Antibiotic
Acne
Candida
Mouth ulcers
Thrush
Veruccae

Cautions: ✗ ★ b i

THYME ~

Keyword: *Bacterial*

Thymus vulgaris

Thyme is distilled from the flowers. A few drops may be used in a bowl of boiling water to relieve nasal congestion.

Physical conditions

Throat infections

Cautions: ✕ b c i P S

This essential oil is best administered by a qualified Aromatherapist.

YLANG YLANG ~

Keyword: *Confidence*

Cananga odorata

Ylang Ylang means flower of flowers. Its exotic fragrance is warming and helpful for instilling confidence.

Psychological conditions

Anger
Aphrodisiac
Detachment
Fear of people, failure
Guilt
Jealousy
Impatience
Irrationality
Irritability
Panic attacks
Secretive
Self confidence
Self esteem
Selfishness
Sensitiveness
Shyness
Stubbornness
Suspiciousness

Cautions: ✕ b i c

9 | Book List

INTRODUCTION
Aromatherapy for Everyone, Robert Tisserand
Aromatherapy for Women, Maggie Tisserand
The Secret of Life & Youth, Marguerite Maury
Herbs & Aromatherapy, Joannah Metcalfe (Culpepper)

READING & REFERENCE
The Art of Aromatherapy, Robert Tisserand
Aromatherapy An A-Z, Patricia Davis
The Fragrant Pharmacy, Valerie Ann Worwood
The Practice of Aromatherapy, Dr Jean Valnet
The Essential Oil Safety Data Manual, Robert Tisserand
Positive Thinking and *You Can Heal your life*, Louise Hay

PHYSICAL CONDITIONS INDEX

ABDOMEN	*Bloated*	Fennel	BC
	Wind	Fennel	BCM
	Colic	Roman Chamomile	BCMbci
	Pains	Lavender	BCMbci
ABSCESS	*External dry*	Lavender	BC
	External weeping	Frankincense	BC
	Mouth	Tea Tree	U
ACNE	*Red face*	Chamomile	BCM
	Pustules	Tea Tree	BCM
	Scarring	Frankincense	BCM
		Lavender	
ADDICTION		Clary Sage, Rose	BMR
ALLERGIES		Rose, Melissa	BCMR
ANTIBIOTICS		Lavender, Tea Tree	BR
APPETITE	*Excessive*	Fennel	BM
	Lack of	Coriander	BM
		Rosemary	
ARTHRITIS	*Redness*	Chamomile	BCM
	Swelling	Juniper	BCM
	Pain with	Lavender	BCM
ASTHMA		Cedarwood	BMIR
		Cypress	
		Eucalyptus	
BALDNESS		Lavender	M
		Rosemary	
BED WETTING		Chamomile	
		Lavender	BMbci
		Cypress	BM
BILIOUS ATTACK	*Nausea*	Peppermint	BIR
		Ginger	
BITES		Lavender	BCN
BLISTERS		Benzoin, Lavender	BC
BLOOD PRESSURE (low)		Hyssop	BM
BLOOD PRESSURE (high)		Hyssop	BM
BOILS		Chamomile	BC
BRONCHITIS	*Generally indicated*	Cedarwood, Pine	BIM
	Cough	Cypress	
	Congestion	Eucalyptus	
	Catarrh	Sandalwood	
BRUISES		Lavender	BC
BURNS		Lavender	BCN
CANDIDA		Tea Tree	BCM
CATARRH		Eucalyptus	BCMIR
		Sandalwood	
CELLULITIS		Cypress	BM
		Fennel	
		Lemon	
CHANGE OF LIFE		Geranium	BM

CHESTINESS	*Dry cough*	Cypress	BCMIR
		Lavender	
		Myrrh, Pine	
	Voice loss	Sandalwood	
CHILDBIRTH		Jasmine	M
CHILBLAINS	*Circulation*	Rosemary	BCM
	Soothing	Sandalwood	
	Itchy and burning	Chamomile	
	Swollen	Lavender	
CHILLINESS	*Cold hands and feet*	Rosemary	BM
	Hugging fires	Rosemary with	
		Frankincense	
	Intense	Ginger	
		Marjoram	
CIRCULATION		Rosemary	BM
COLDS	*Shivering,*	Cinnamon	BMR
	Flu-like	Eucalyptus,	
	symptoms	Ginger	
	Frequent sneezing	Cypress	BMIR
	Runny nose	Eucalyptus	
COLIC		Chamomile	CMbci
		Fennel	CM
		Cardamon	
CONSTIPATION		Rosemary	BM
		Black Pepper	
CORNS		Lemon	B
COUGHS	*Dry*	Cypress	BMIR
	Voice loss	Sandalwood	
CRAMP	*Recurring*	Juniper	BM
	After exercise	Rosemary and	
		Marjoram	
		with Lemongrass	
CUTS		Lavender	BCNc
			bi (Always dilute)
CYSTITIS	*General*	Juniper	
		Sandalwood	B
	Pain on passing water	Lavender	
	With a temperature	Eucalyptus	
DANDRUFF	*Oily scalp*	Cypress	☐
		Cedarwood	
	Dry scalp	Rosemary	
DERMATITIS		Chamomile	BCM
		Geranium	(Check for any
		Lavender	irritants e.g.
			detergents)
EARACHE		Lavender	Cic
ECZEMA	*Skin cracked*	Lavender with	
	and weeping	Frankincense	
	Sensitive to touch	Geranium with	
		Lavender	BC
	Itching	Chamomile	BCM
	Burning and hot	Chamomile	

Condition		Oil	Method
EXHAUSTION		Clary Sage with Lavender Orange	BMR
FAINTING		Basil, Rosemary	I
FLATULENCE		Fennel	BCM
	Excess eating	Fennel	BC
	With wind	Fennel	BC
HAEMORRHOIDS		Cypress, Frankincense	BM
HANGOVER		Rose, Juniper Rosemary	B
HAYFEVER		Juniper, Rose	B
HEADACHE	*Tension*	Lavender	BCM
	Travel sickness	Peppermint	BCI
	With a cold	Eucalyptus	BCMI
	Sinus congestion	Basil	BMI
	Migraine	Lavender Rosemary	BCI (Massage is also helpful though should not be attempted whilst experiencing the migraine)
HOARSENESS	*Laryngitis*	Sandalwood with Lavender	BMR
	Straining vocal chords		BMR
HOT FLUSHES		Chamomile with Geranium	BM
HYPERTENSION		Hyssop	BM
HYPOTENSION		Hyssop	BM
IMMUNE SYSTEM STIMULANT		Lavender	BMR
INDIGESTION		Fennel Cardamon	BM
INFLUENZA		Cinnamon Black Pepper Ginger	BCM (Combined with Jasmine has been found very effective in early stages of flu)
INSECT BITES		Lavender	BCN
INSECT REPELLENT		Lemongrass Lavender	BMR
INSOMNIA	*Restless in bed*	Lavender	BMR★
	Feels overtired	Clary Sage	BMR
	Nightmares	Frankincense	
ITCHY SKIN		Peppermint	B (Use one drop in the bath with Lavender)
JOINTS	*Swollen*	Chamomile Juniper	BCM
	Painful	Lavender	
	Rheumatic	Juniper	
LARYNGITIS	*General*	Sandalwood with	BMR

40

LARYNGITIS – *cont*		Lavender	
	Loss of voice		
	Tickling cough		
LICE	*Body*	Geranium	BC
	Head		□
LIGAMENTS	*Painful from over-exertion*	Lemongrass and Rosemary	BM
METABOLISM STIMULANT		Sage	B
MIGRAINE	*Allergy*	Rose, Juniper	BM (Do not massage
	Tension	Lavender	whilst migraine is active)
MUSCLE ACHES	*After exercise*	Lemongrass and Rosemary	BM (May also be used before exercise)
	With fever	Black Pepper	B
	Convalescing	Cypress and Rosemary	BM
NAUSEA	*With migraine*	Lavender	
		Peppermint	B○
	From overeating	Fennel	
	Travel sickness	Peppermint	BCI○
NECK	*Stiff*	Lavender	BCMR
NETTLE RASH		Chamomile	BC
NEURALGIA		Peppermint	C
NOSEBLEED		Cypress, Frankincense	C
		Lavender	
OEDEMA		Juniper	BCM
OVERWEIGHT		Fennel	BM
		Patchouli	
OVERWORK		Clary Sage	BM (These essential
		Lavender	oils encourage a good night's rest)
		Rosemary	B (A stimulating bath after a good night's rest)
PERIODS	*Heavy*	Cypress	BCM
	Irregular	Geranium	
		Melissa	
	Scanty	Juniper	
PMT	*Tender breasts*	Geranium	BM
	Depression	Bergamot	BMR
	Irritable	Lavender	
	Water retention	Juniper	BM
	Weepy	Rose	BM
	Moody	Geranium	BM
PREGNANCY			

(see special directions for using Essential oils and Essential oils to avoid at this time)

	Breast-feeding	Fennel	M (Massage after
		Geranium	feeding and wash before next feed)
	Refreshing	Geranium	B
		Lavender	

PREGNANCY– *cont*		Rose	
	Morning sickness	Cardamon	R
		Ginger	
	Pre-birth	Ylang Ylang	BR
		Sandalwood	
		Rosewood	
	Birth	Jasmine	R
		Lavender	CM (Use to ease
		Clary Sage	CM birth pains)
	Post-birth	Frankincense	BR
		Lavender	
		Neroli	
		Bergamot	BM
	Depression	Geranium, Jasmine	
	Sleep-disturbed	Lavender	(A couple of drops
			on the pillow at night)
PSORIASIS		Bergamot	BCM
		Geranium	
		Lavender	
RESPIRATORY TRACT		Eucalyptus	BCIM
		Pine, Tea Tree	
RHEUMATOID		Chamomile	
ARTHRITIS		Juniper	BCM
		Ginger	
		Lavender	
SHIVERING	*From cold*	Marjoram	BM
		Rosemary	
	Flu-like	Cinnamon	B
SICKNESS	*Travel*	Peppermint	BCI○
	Stomach pains	Black Pepper	BCM
		Peppermint	
		Lavender	
	Alcohol	Juniper, Rose	
	After overeating	Fennel	
SINUSITIS	*Head pain*	Eucalyptus	BCIM
		Lavender	
	Congestion	Basil	
	Catarrh	Eucalyptus	
		Sandalwood	
SKIN	*Blotches*	Geranium	BCM
	Broken veins	Neroli	BC
	Burning sensation	Lavender	BC
	Burns	Lavender	BCN
	Chapped	Benzoin	BM
		Sandalwood	
	Cracked	Frankincense	
		Patchouli	
	Weeping eczema	Lavender	BC
	Dry	Geranium with	
		Sandalwood	BM
	Inflamed	Chamomile	BC
	Itchy	Lavender	BCM

SKIN – *cont*	*Mature*	Juniper, Rose	BM
	Normal	Geranium	BM
	Oily	Cedarwood	BM
	Sensitive	Chamomile, Rose	BCM
SPRAINS	*Bruising*	Lavender	C
	Joints/Tendons	Chamomile	
STINGS	*Insect*	Lavender	BCN
STOMACH ACHE		Peppermint	BCM
KIDNEY STONES		Juniper	BM
SUNBURN		Lavender	BC
TEETHING		Chamomile	bci
TENDONS	*Over-exertion*	Rosemary	BM
	Painful	Lavender	
	Rheumatism	Juniper	
THROAT	*Sore*	Lavender	BCM
		Sandalwood	
	Dry/Burning	Lavender	
THROAT	*Infections*	Tea Tree	M
		Thyme	
THRUSH		Tea Tree	B
TINNITUS	*Sensitive*	Lavender	CM
	Nausea	Peppermint	
	Catarrh worsens	Sandalwood	
TIREDNESS	*Mental*	Rosemary	BM (Relaxing oils
	Physical	Rosemary	BM may be used to obtain a good night's rest)
TOOTHACHE		Clove, Peppermint	CM
TRAVEL	*Sickness*	Peppermint	BCIM
	Restlessness	Lavender	
	With fear	Bergamot	
		Chamomile	BCIMbci
	Sensitivity to movement	Peppermint	BCIMc
URINATION	*Burning/Painful*	Juniper and Sandalwood	BM
	Frequent	Cypress	BM
VARICOSE VEINS		Cypress, Lavender	BC (Patience is required. Treat very gently.)
VOICE LOSS	*Hoarseness from overuse with Laryngitis*	Sandalwood Lavender	BCM
VERUCCAS		Tea Tree	U
WARTS		Lemon	U
WINDBURN		Lavender	B
WOUNDS		Lavender	BCN

PSYCHOLOGICAL CONDITIONS INDEX

The essential oils listed under this heading may be used in baths, massages or as room fragrancers.

ANXIETY		Bergamot
ANGER		Ylang Ylang
APATHY	*Emotional/Spiritual*	Jasmine
	Mental/Physical	Rosemary
APHRODISIAC		Jasmine, Ylang Ylang
APPREHENSION		Frankincense, Patchouli
ATTACHMENT		Geranium, Rose
ATTENTION SPAN	*Short*	Basil
BEREAVEMENT	*Shock*	Neroli
	Prolonged grief	Frankincense
	Lost in past	Rose
BITTERNESS		Grapefruit
BRAIN	*Tired*	Basil
	Dread of effort	Sandalwood
	Dull	Rosemary
	Bad memory	Rosemary
BOREDOM		Lemongrass
CLARITY		Grapefruit, Rosemary
CLAUSTROPHOBIA		Clary Sage, Frankincense
COMPULSIVENESS		Cajuput, Clary Sage, Patchouli
CONCENTRATION	*Lack of*	Basil, Lemongrass
CONFIDENCE	*Lack of*	Jasmine
CONFUSION		Cardamon, Grapefruit
COURAGE		Frankincense
CYNICISM		Cajuput, Sandalwood
DAYDREAMING	*Excessive*	Camphor, Rosewood
DEPRESSION		Bergamot, Clary Sage
DESPONDENCY		Bergamot, Grapefruit
DISTANT, DETACHED FEELING		Jasmine, Ylang Ylang
DISORIENTATION		Cajuput, Rosemary
	With shock	Neroli
DREAMS	*Recurrent*	Clary Sage, Sandalwood
	Nightmares	Frankincense
EMOTIONAL EXPRESSION		Jasmine
ENVY		Grapefruit, Rose
EXHAUSTION	*Mental*	Basil, Rosemary
	Rest following	Lavender
FEAR	*Following a fright*	Frankincense, Lavender
	Terror	Frankincense, Rose
	Coming events	Jasmine, Sandalwood
	Of failure	Lavender, Sandalwood
	Of people	Lavender, Ylang Ylang
	Stagefright	Lavender, Ylang Ylang
	Unknown origin	Frankincense, Rose
FRUSTRATION		Grapefruit
GRIEF		Hyssop, Rose

GUILT		Ylang Ylang
HOSTILITY		Clary Sage, Marjoram, Ylang Ylang
HUMILITY		Melissa, Sandalwood
HYSTERIA		Neroli, Lavender
HYPERACTIVITY		Clary Sage, Lavender, Marjoram
INDECISIVENESS		Grapefruit, Rosemary
IMPATIENCE		Lavender, Ylang Ylang
INSOMNIA		Clary Sage, Lavender
INSECURITY		Frankincense, Lavender, Sandalwood
INTUITION		Sandalwood
IRRATIONAL	*Personality*	Lavender, Ylang Ylang
	Thoughts	Lavender, Marjoram
IRRITABILITY	*Jealousy*	Grapefruit, Ylang Ylang
	Fright	Neroli, Frankincense
	Anger	Ylang, Ylang
	Grief	Rose, Sandalwood
	Impulsiveness	Chamomile
	Short temperedness	Lavender, Sandalwood
JEALOUSY		Cypress, Jasmine, Ylang Ylang
LETHARGY		Juniper, Rosemary
LISTLESSNESS		Clary Sage, Sandalwood
LONELINESS		Benzoin, Melissa
MEMORY		Cajuput, Rosemary, Basil
MENTAL	*Calmness*	Lavender, Sandalwood
	Clarity	Cajuput, Grapefruit, Rosemary
	Stimulation	Basil, Peppermint, Rosemary
MONDAY MORNING FEELING		Rosemary combined with one of the Citrus oils e.g. Bergamot
MOOD SWINGS		Geranium, Lavender
NEGATIVE THOUGHTS		Bergamot, Clary Sage, Lavender
NERVES	*Worry about future*	Camphor, Melissa, Sandalwood
	Worry about past	Grapefruit, Frankincense, Rose
NIGHTMARES		Frankincense
OBSESSION		Bergamot, Clary Sage, Lavender
OVER-ANALYTICAL		Clary Sage, Jasmine
OVERWORK	*Mental strain*	Clary Sage, Marjoram, Neroli
	Nervous exhaustion	Clary Sage, Lavender, Lemongrass, Neroli
PARANOIA		Lavender, Frankincense, Rosewood
PERSEVERANCE IN DIFFICULT CIRCUMSTANCES		Frankincense, Sandalwood
PROCRASTINATION		Cajuput, Grapefruit, Sandalwood
PROTECTION		Juniper, Rosemary, Sandalwood
REJUVENATING		Frankincense
RELAXATION		Clary Sage, Lavender, Marjoram, Rosewood
RESTLESSNESS	*Active mind*	Chamomile, Lavender
	With exhaustion	Clary Sage, Neroli
	Apprehension	Lavender, Rosewood
PANIC ATTACKS		Frankincense, Lavender
RIGIDITY		Geranium, Jasmine, Ylang Ylang
REGRET		Bergamot, Rose
SADNESS		Benzoin, Jasmine, Rose

SECURITY	Frankincense, Lavender, Sandalwood
SECRETIVENESS	Jasmine, Ylang Ylang
SELF-ACCEPTANCE	Ginger
SELF-AWARENESS	Rose
SELF-CENTREDNESS	Rose, Sandalwood
SELF-CONFIDENCE	Bergamot, Ylang Ylang
SELF-CRITICAL	Frankincense, Sandalwood, Ylang Ylang
SELF-ESTEEM	Sandalwood, Ylang Ylang
STABILITY	Frankincense, Rosewood
SELFISHNESS	Lemon or Orange with Ylang Ylang
SENSITIVITY	Juniper, Sandalwood, Ylang Ylang
SHOCK	Melissa, Neroli
SHYNESS	Bergamot, Jasmine, Ylang Ylang
SLUGGISHNESS	Lemon, Cypress, Rosemary
STAGE FRIGHT	Lavender, Ylang Ylang
STRESS	Cedarwood, Clary Sage, Neroli
STUBBORNNESS	Orange, Ylang Ylang
SULKINESS	Clary Sage, Lemongrass
SUSPICIOUSNESS	Melissa, Frankincense, Ylang Ylang
TOO EXTROVERT/INTROVERT	Geranium, Lavender, Jasmine
TOO TALKATIVE	Cypress
UNDISCIPLINED	Basil, Frankincense
TANTRUM	Chamomile
WORRY	Chamomile, Lavender

OTHER BOOKS FROM AMBERWOOD PUBLISHING ARE:

Aromatherapy Lexicon — The Essential Reference by Geoff Lyth and Sue Charles is a colourful, fun way to learn about Aromatherapy. £4.99.

Aromatherapy - The Baby Book by Marion Del Gaudio Mak. An easy to follow guide to massage for the infant or child. £3.99

Aromatherapy — For Stress Management by Christine Westwood. Covering the use of essential oils for everyday stress-related problems. £3.50.

Aromatherapy — For Healthy Legs and Feet by Christine Westwood. A guide to the use of essential oils for the treatment of legs and feet. £2.99.

Aromatherapy — Simply For You by Marion Del Gaudio Mak. A clear, simple and comprehensive guide to Aromatherapy for beginners. £1.99.

Aromatherapy — A Nurses Guide by Ann Percival SRN. The ultimate, safe, lay guide to the natural benefits of Aromatherapy. Including recipes and massage techniques for many medical conditions and a quick reference chart. £2.99.

Aromatherapy — A Nurses Guide for Women by Ann Percival SRN. Concentrates on women's health for all ages. Including sections on PMT, menopause, infertility, cellulite. £2.99.

Aromatherapy — Essential Oils in Colour by Rosemary Caddy Bsc Hons, ARCS MISP is a unique book depicting the chemistry of Essential oils. £9.99.

Aroma Science — The Chemistry & Bioactivity of Essential Oils by Dr Maria Lis-Balchin. With a comprehensive list of the Oils and scientific analysis. Includes sections on the sense of smell and the history of Aromatherapy. £4.99.

Plant Medicine — A Guide for Home Use (New Edition) by Charlotte Mitchell MNIMH. A guide to home use giving an insight into the wonderful healing qualities of plants. £2.99.

Woman Medicine — Vitex Agnus Castus by Simon Mills MA, FNIMH. The story of the herb that has been used for centuries in the treatment of women's problems. £2.99.

Ancient Medicine — Ginkgo Biloba (New Edition) by Dr Desmond Corrigan BSc(Pharms), MA, Phd, FLS, FPSI. Improved memory, circulation and concentration are associated with Ginkgo and explained in this book. £2.99.

Indian Medicine — The Immune System by Dr Desmond Corrigan BSc(Pharms), MA, Phd, FLS, FPSI. An intriguing account of the history of the plant called Echinacea and its power to influence the immune system. £2.99.

Herbal Medicine for Sleep & Relaxation by Dr Desmond Corrigan BSc(Pharms), MA, PhD, FLS, FPSI. A guide to the natural sedatives as an alternative to orthodox drug therapies, drawing on the latest medical research, presented in an easy reference format. £2.99.

Herbal First Aid by Andrew Chevallier BA, MNIMH. A beautifully clear reference book of natural remedies and general first aid in the home. £2.99.

Natural Taste – Herbal Teas, A Guide for Home Use by Andrew Chevallier BA, MNIMH. Contains a comprehensive compendium of Herbal Teas gives information on how to make it, its benefits, history and folklore. £3.50.

Garlic– How Garlic Protects Your Heart by Prof E. Ernst MD, PhD. Used as a medicine for over 4500 years, this book examines the latest scientific evidence supporting Garlic's effect in reducing cardiovascular disease, the Western World's number one killer. £3.99.

Phytotherapy-50 Vital Herbs by Andrew Chevallier, the most popular Medicinal herbs with uses and advice written by an expert-£6.99.

Insomnia – Doctor I Can't Sleep by Dr Adrian Williams FRCP. Written by one of the world's leading sleep experts, Dr Williams explains the phenomenon of sleep and sleeping disorders and gives advice on treatment. With 25% of the adult population reporting difficulties sleeping – this book will be essential reading for many. £2.99.

Signs & Symptoms of Vitamin Deficiency by Dr Leonard Mervyn BSc, PhD, C.Chem, FRCS. A home guide for self diagnosis which explains and assesses Vitamin Therapy for the prevention of a wide variety of diseases and illnesses. £2.99.

Causes & Prevention of Vitamin Deficiency by Dr Leonard Mervyn BSc, PhD, C.Chem, FRCS. A home guide to the Vitamin content of foods and the depletion caused by cooking, storage and processing. It includes advice for those whose needs are increased due to lifestyle, illness etc. £2.99.

Eyecare Eyewear – For Better Vision by Mark Rossi Bsc, MBCO. A complete guide to eyecare and eyewear including an assessment of the types of spectacles and contact lenses available and the latest corrective surgical procedures. £3.99.

Arthritis and Rheumatism by Dr John Cosh FRCP, MD. Covers all forms of Arthritis, its affects and the treatments available. £4.95.